BEING
HUMAN

BEING HUMAN

THE YAMAS & NIYAMAS

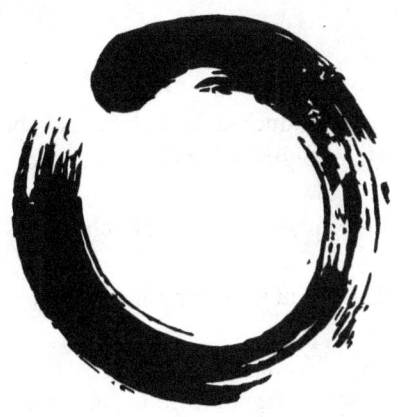

An exploration of yoga's ethical principles
from the complicated lens of human existence

SARA ADAMS

Book design and production by Columbus Publishing Lab
www.ColumbusPublishingLab.com

Author photo courtesy of Bob Cervas

Copyright © 2021 by Sara Adams

www.BeingHuman.yoga
https://www.instagram.com/beinghuman.yoga

All rights reserved. This book, or parts thereof, may not be reproduced in any form without permission.

Paperback ISBN: 978-1-63337-542-0
E-book ISBN: 978-1-63337-543-7
LCCN: 2021917667

1 3 5 7 9 10 8 6 4 2

CONTENTS

The Gray 1

The Yamas 9
Ahimsa | Less Harm 11
Satya | Truth 23
Asteya | Non-Stealing 35
Brahmacharya | Enough 45
Aparigraha | Softening Attachments 53

The Niyamas 63
Saucha | Purification 65
Santosha | Contentment 75
Tapas | Discipline 85
Svadhyaya | Self-Study 95
Isvara Pranidhana | Acceptance 105

The Beginning 115

The Gray

"I realized that I don't have to be perfect. All I have to do is show up and enjoy the messy, imperfect, and beautiful journey of my life. It's a trip more wonderful than I could have imagined."
—Kerry Washington

I WAS IN THE MIDDLE OF WRITING THIS BOOK at **the** start of 2020, and damn was I in a flow. Then...well, you know the rest. The world was facing both a global pandemic and a long-overdue cry for racial justice. From society's perspective, it was an emotionally heavy time. In my small corner of the world, I was facing my own emotional heaviness—the end of my marriage. Needless to say, the writing took a back seat.

Fast forward to late November of that same year. I was settling in to my divorce apartment. It was the first time I'd ever lived by myself. Making a space all your own is something truly special, and mine needed a bookcase. I spent hours searching, finally deciding on one I hoped would be the perfect fit. It even came with in-room delivery, which was a huge plus considering the nightmarish stairs that led to my second-floor apartment. The delivery driver arrived with two boxes.

"Two boxes for one bookcase?" I asked him.

"Yep," he said, "I have two going to this address."

Two boxes? That thing was going to be a bitch to put together, but I was up for the challenge!

I decided to tackle it that Saturday, only to find out that both boxes weren't for the bookcase. The other box contained a desk. A desk I hadn't ordered, because I had no need for a desk. I didn't work from home, and there wasn't a place for it in my apartment. I couldn't, in good conscience, keep it, so I called to tell the manufacturer that there had been a mistake. The representative said that they might not want it back, and if they didn't call me in two weeks, the desk was mine. Two weeks and no phone call later, I had a desk to get rid of. I still had no need for it, so I tried to sell it online. I even tried to entice people by telling them I'd donate the money to a charity of their choosing. After all, I hadn't spent any money. Why not do some good for free? Weeks went by with no takers. Zero.

Fast forward another few weeks. I was feeling optimistic about the new year and starting to think about what 2021 might bring. I was also annoyed that there was still a huge box sitting idly in my nice, tidy apartment. Then it dawned on me...maybe this really *was* my desk. I was finally getting back to a healthier mental space after everything that had happened in 2020. I was starting to remember things that once brought me joy, and had even thought about my book a time or two. So I shifted my perspective and decided that it was a gift from the universe — a sign that it was time to start writing again. I spent an entire day building my new desk and rearranging my apartment to accommodate it. I'll never know why I thought I didn't have the space for that thing, because it fit perfectly once I opened myself up to the idea of it. With my desk nestled nicely in the corner of my living room I started writing again, and this time I actually finished.

Does life always work out with such poetic serendipity? No, of course not. Also, yes, it absolutely does! Life creates unmatched beauty *and* brings overwhelming pain. It gives us the good and the bad, often all at once. You can choose to gaze through either lens. The trick is to gaze through them both simultaneously. That's what I'm here to share. The *ands*—that gray space where all of life actually exists.

Back in 2015, I completed my 200-hour yoga teacher training. There was a lot more philosophical discussion than I expected, and I was loving it! My eyes were opening to yoga beyond heated rooms and headstands. For the first time in my life, I felt like my many guarded layers were pulled back, and all that was left was my truest self. I had found a community of like-minded individuals who would be there to champion my journey, just like I would champion theirs. I absorbed all of this incredible knowledge through the lens of my life so far. Take note: That lens was built with society's black and white extremes. It was built with immediate gratification and the misconception that failure was unacceptable. It was also built with the pressure to accomplish as much as possible while always being positive and helpful.

Throughout our philosophical discussions, I found two ethical practices to be particularly impactful, which is why we're here. But let's back up a bit first. In yogic philosophy, the Yoga Sutras of Patanjali are regarded as the foundational framework for its practice. Patanjali identifies the eight Limbs of Yoga, which include:

Yamas: restraints
Niyamas: inner observances
Asana: posture
Pranayama: breath
Pratyahara: sensory withdrawal
Dharana: concentration
Dhyana: meditation
Samadhi: enlightenment

The disciplined practice of all eight is said to create wholeness in one's life. The Yamas and Niyamas were the two that really took hold for me. As I explored each Yama and

Niyama, I found it almost poetic how they played so well off of each other. Because their teachings are so connected, they are commonly studied in conjunction with one another. While they do intertwine, each principle includes a specific subset of practices.

The Yamas are an external practice of how we interact with the world and its people. The five are:

Ahimsa: non-harm
Satya: truth
Asteya: non-stealing
Brahmacharya: non-excess
Aparigraha: non-attachment

Niyamas are an inside job, the internal work toward self-exploration and living with purpose and ease. They include:

Saucha: purification
Santosha: contentment
Tapas: discipline
Svadhyaya: self-study
Isvara Pranidhana: surrender

I remember thinking that if I focused enough time on these practices, I would be happy for the rest of my life. And that's the goal, right? Constant, uninterrupted happiness? How could I not fall in love with ten simple ideas that would help me achieve the very thing I'd always wanted? It wasn't until I became very unhappy (right before and throughout my divorce) that I started to see how unrealistic that expectation was. I understood that life could be a bit of a rollercoaster, but mine had always been in the kiddie section. After my spiritual enlightenment via teacher training, certainly I was exempt from experiencing any extremely difficult emotions? At the very least, I was properly equipped to handle them with ease and grace. Right?

Life came along to humble me, as it so often does. Everything I was doing to cope was a contradiction of these practices, which felt like failure. That sense of failure quickly turned into guilt and a lack of self-worth. Why was I feeling guilty for my behaviors when I wouldn't hesitate to give others grace? That's when the dots started to connect. It became clear that learning these concepts through my Midwestern point of view had been less than helpful. My standard of self was established with a high bar from a young age. When I came to the yoga classroom, I reinforced that bar with everything I was learning. In essence, while I found my best self, I stopped accepting any other versions of me.

I eventually saw that I had brought my black-and-white lens of extremes into my study of the Yamas and Niyamas. It wasn't the teachings themselves; it was how I was viewing them. I excluded any wiggle room for imperfection and real life. Non-harm, contentment, non-attachment. They all seemed so absolute. I was either doing it, or I wasn't. If I wasn't, I was failing. I decided to explore these teachings in a way that allowed for more *real* life. Less extremes, more gray.

Initially, I met myself with a lot of resistance. Once I gave myself permission to be human, I was actually able to move forward. And I am human. A very simple, complicated, ordinary, unique human. I don't have a master's degree in psychology, and I haven't spent decades studying ancient yogic texts. I'm a 200-hour-trained yoga teacher with a bachelor's degree in marketing who works a nine-to-five as an HR professional. Oh, and sometimes I teach yoga, but not always. Basically, I'm a pretty regular person with a pretty regular life. I am also naturally curious about people: why we do what we do, and all of our wonderful complexities. I've spent hours reflecting on the Yamas and Niyamas, both as my best self and at my most vulnerable. I'm here to share the truths I've found on either end and in the middle.

The Yamas
yah·muhs

"Your impact on the world is significant whether or not you are aware of it, and even whether or not you desire it."
—Gary Zukav

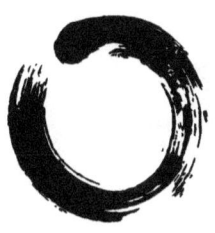

Ahimsa - अहिंसा
uh·hims·uh
~~Non-Harm~~
Less Harm

EARLY INTO THE PANDEMIC, I HAD TO WORK FROM home for two weeks after being exposed to COVID-19 during a meeting. Most of my inner circle was either already working from home, laid off, or furloughed. I was the oddball who had to keep going to a physical office, so I was actually a little relieved to have what was becoming a "normal" experience. That first morning I started setting things up in the bedroom. My husband had already been working from home for a while, so he was set up in our office. As I unpacked my laptop and notebook, I thought about how the next couple of weeks would be similar to retirement, where we would both be home together all day. My next thought took the wind right out of me. *I don't want that for my future.* Sure, I'd experienced moments of doubt throughout our fifteen-year relationship, but never anything that felt so certain. It was a true moment of intuition, one that I would spend weeks trying to un-feel. That's the thing about intuition. In the quickest of instants it tells us everything we need to know about what's in our heart, but we only hear it when we're ready to listen.

I wasn't ready to hear it, but I couldn't make it go away either. Was I just being impulsive? Was I just processing a million complex pandemic emotions, and this was how they were showing up? Or did I know, deep down, that I didn't want to wake up a seventy-year-old woman who had nothing to talk about with her husband because he never got to know her? My mind was flooded with thoughts and emotions that I was frantically trying to rationalize.

During all of this, I was struggling with the concept of non-harm. Ahimsa had become a foundational part of my life. I composted, ate a mostly vegan diet, positioned myself in a profession where I could influence actual change for people who really needed it, and was annoyingly tedious about recycling. Now I was faced with a decision that would cause harm no matter what. Obviously leaving would cause harm, and so would staying. I was hung up on the *non*. Finally, I told myself that if no harm wasn't an option, I'd have to settle for less. *Less harm.* The idea felt freeing. That subtle shift in language opened up a level of permission that I had been desperately searching for.

Rationally, I knew it was impossible to never cause any harm in my life. Emotionally, it was extremely difficult to admit that I had to.

The thing is, most of us cause harm every single day. Our brains help us ignore things that are hard to digest, even once we are aware of them. Our brain also decides which things will plague us with guilt. I didn't think twice about the several online orders coming to my house each week that were manufactured inhumanely in China, picked and packed by warehouse workers on their sixth consecutive ten-hour shift, and delivered by drowsy drivers in gas-guzzling trucks. But you'd better believe I'd pull a water bottle out of my coworker's trash can and recycle it. Does that mean I'm an awful human? Of course not. It means I'm a normal human. It also means that our society has normalized harm through millions of small actions that add up to something much larger. But more on all that later.

One of my core values is to always assume positive intent, both for others and for myself. When things feel personal, this value leaves space for me to realize that they usually aren't. If you're here doing this work, I bet you're not actively trying to hurt people. Still, there will be plenty of times when you do, even when you didn't mean to. Trusting our positive intentions helps with accountability. Sometimes we realize that our actions will cause harm, and sometimes we don't. When we know, it's easier to address the harm we've caused with empathy and kindness. When we don't know, we can become defensive about our good intentions and dismiss another's experience of us. The trick is to pause. If we can pause and accept someone else's truth, we cause less harm. We can't undo the initial hurt, but taking accountability prevents additional harm that our reaction may cause. Pause. Apologize. Learn.

We have the opportunity to practice Ahimsa toward others every day. It shows up when we don't publicly call out our coworker who's been slacking off, and instead have a one-on-one conversation with them to see if they are okay. It shows up when we offer support instead of solutions to our friend struggling with addiction, or when we are understanding instead of angry with the barista who got our order wrong. It's as simple as seeing the humanity in others and behaving in a way that embraces all of the complex possibilities that could be weighing on them. Accept that others are experiencing life in a way that you may or may not understand, and let that be okay.

As we move deeper into the work, Ahimsa takes on a more proactive role. Remember those millions of small actions that add up to something bigger? That's how problems like climate change, systemic racism, and many others take shape. It's also how they improve. Get curious about your passions and help those movements in the ways you're able. No one way is right or better, and every action has value. Sure, you could live on a small plot of land in a home with 100 percent renewable energy, growing all of your own food and repairing your second-hand clothes as they become tattered. That would be a tremendous and admirable effort in the name of less harm. For most of us, the work comes in baby steps. We can do small things often, and that will have a big impact.

If you keep increasing your awareness, new ways to influence change will present themselves. Maybe you want to buy less fast fashion and introduce your family to Meatless Monday. Maybe you work for a corporation that is a major environmental polluter, but that career affords you the ability to cook locally sourced organic foods and donate money to agencies that are driving important social justice movements forward. When you stay curious and keep learning, you find new opportunities for less harm. When you forgive yourself and others for the ways we all still cause harm, you clear the path to continue forward.

I remember when I first started embracing Ahimsa years ago. I was excited to make vegan food tasty and was slowly switching to cruelty-free household products. I had created some bomb-ass recipes and was proud to produce more recycling than trash. There's a lot to be said for early wins. They give us the confidence to keep going, which leads to that curiosity to do more. It's why we're more successful when we start small.

Eventually, we have to do the inner work, which tends to be more difficult. Here's the thing: You'll spend more time with your own thoughts than you will with anything or anyone else. Your inner monologue shapes your life, and everything inside projects outward. The problem is that most of us reach adulthood projecting our expansive collection of low self-image, unearned guilt, and constant self-doubt. Let me tell you what—this collection is almost as lame as my Beanie Babies from the '90s, and definitely less valuable. We end up with years of shit to unlearn about ourselves, because we learned false truths that others projected onto us, which had first been projected onto them. And so on and so on. If we want to, we can break the cycle.

It starts with awareness. You have to listen closely to your thoughts. How are you speaking to yourself? Are you celebrating your wins or questioning if they're even yours to celebrate? Do you love who you see in the mirror, or do you say hurtful things to yourself? Be honest about what you are saying to you, and be honest about how you feel when you hear those words.

After you've learned to listen, you can work on accepting your thoughts as they are. Give yourself permission to accept them without worrying about changing them or beating yourself up for saying them in the first place. Saying more mean things to yourself about the mean things you're already saying to yourself perpetuates the cycle.

Once you've accepted them, you can start to change the narrative. For me, it's most helpful to imagine saying to a loved one the things I tell myself. I would never tell my best friend "everything you like is stupid and uninteresting" or "you might as well quit because you never really finish anything anyways." The thought makes me cringe. And it should, because those are really shitty things to say to someone. Still, I said them to myself time and time again for many years. You can change your own narrative by not saying anything to yourself when you'd normally say something critical. You can take it a step further and change the monologue to something positive and supportive. I still catch myself being mean to me sometimes. Funny enough, when that happens, I'm usually also being short with others. Everything inside projects outward. When you cultivate less harm toward yourself, it naturally ripples.

The most important work you'll ever do is on yourself. I know how hard that work is, and I know how valuable it is. I've done it, am doing it, and will always be doing it. As life unfolds, you'll get to know yourself at many different levels of stress. Let's say it's a ten-point scale. At a one, you're calm and clear. At ten, you're barely keeping it together.

Practicing Ahimsa changes depending on that level, which is normal and okay! At my ones and twos, I feel amazing. My interactions with others are effortless; my body feels light and full of energy; I feel good about my carbon footprint; my relationship with self is at its best. At my nines and tens, I'm a bitch to myself and others. I'm definitely not concerned with activism or what the fuck I'm eating, and you can usually find me crying behind the credenza in my office.

When extreme stress or life-changing events kick us into those nines and tens, sometimes we barely have capacity to get through our days. Less harm during those times is trusting that you're doing your best and knowing that you've built a solid foundation of goodness that will catch you once you heal. It's important to accept that you'll veer off your path and also to trust that you'll find it again. Remember to forgive yourself for being human along the way.

The Work

I am definitely a type-A person at my core, but I have tons of type-B sprinkles on top. Basically, I need structure to get things done, but I need my time to daydream, too. I'm also an optimistic realist. I think that life is overwhelming sometimes and great other times, and we never know how long each cycle will last. That's how I have decided to structure the work around each Yama and Niyama.

After each topic, you'll get to explore each Yama and Niyama for yourself. Each time, we will start with a check-in to see how you're feeling and what life is throwing at you. Your answer will point you toward specific prompts that will help you do the work in a manageable way considering your life's circumstances.

Just know that there is no timeline for this work, nor is there a destination. Maybe you read this book cover-to-cover in a single day. Maybe you spend an entire month exploring each practice in depth. However it shows up in your life currently, I recommend revisiting this section for each Yama and Niyama as life cycles between overwhelming, great, and in between. The work looks different at each cycle. It doesn't mean that the work you do while life is great is more valuable than the work you do when life is overwhelming. It all becomes part of your journey and is equally important to explore. So let's check in.

How does life feel right now?

1. I feel overwhelmed. Life is coming at me hard and I feel like I can barely keep it together.
2. I feel okay. I have some things I'm working through, and my to-do list is longer than I like it to be. But overall I'm doing fine.
3. I feel great! My heart and mind are wide open, and my stress level is manageable.

Next, find your work:

THE WORK AT OVERWHELMED

Forgive yourself for something you've done that caused harm.

Let this be enough work for now.

THE WORK AT OKAY

Explore some simple efforts that cause less harm and enjoy the early wins! Afterwards, ask yourself, "Is it possible to do this more often?" Here are some ideas if you'd like a jumping-off point:

- Skip buying the $8 clearance shirt
- Eat vegan for a day
- Buy an eco-friendly multi-use cleaner instead of multiple single-purpose ones
- Get your boots resoled instead of buying a new pair
- See if you can go one day without creating any waste
- Wash and reuse/recycle that plastic carryout container you'd normally trash (Remember to check your local guidelines first!)

What cause are you passionate about? What can you do to support them more this week? Longer term?

THE WORK AT GREAT

Identify a negative perception that you can unlearn about yourself. After you find it, do the work. Listen to the thought when it comes up. Next, accept the thought as it is. Finally, work to change the narrative. Spend all the time you need with this one.

When the opportunity presents itself, hold space for someone else's experience of you. If you learn that you've hurt them in some way, pause, apologize, and learn.

YOUR WORK

Each time, we will close out the work with an invitation to explore each Yama and Niyama on your own. I can only share my experiences from the perspective of my life so far. And I can only pose questions that have been meaningful to me during this work. Your personal exploration is so much more important than anything I can share or ask. This part is all for you.

Explore Ahimsa on your own. Notice what resonates. Notice the points of resistance. Notice your body's physical reaction as you explore. Let yourself get curious about what comes up.

Satya - सत्य
suh·ty·uh
Truth

I USED TO THINK TRUTH WAS A SIMPLE CONCEPT. Something was true or it wasn't. I was being honest or I was lying. Black and white and simple. Of course, life is more complex than that. The *truth* is, most situations have many truths. Even when we think we are telling *the* truth, we are still just telling *our* truth.

Recently, an employee came to my office to share a concern. Let's pretend her name is Natalie. (Already a lie in our section on truth!) Natalie told me that one of her coworkers was being rude to her. She was going through a rough patch and had started crying at her work station a few times. Sometimes she had to leave to collect herself in the bathroom. Natalie told me that her coworker had pointed at her and told the supervisor to send her home. She knew this was true because she saw this coworker go over to their supervisor and point at her. A few minutes later, the supervisor asked Natalie if she wanted to go home since she was visibly upset. Natalie was extremely distraught and didn't feel like she was welcome at work anymore. It was my job to find out why this had all happened, so I started talking to the others involved.

When I spoke to her coworker, she told me that she didn't know who Natalie was. When I asked her about the pointing, she explained that she had been pointing at two other employees working near Natalie for a completely different reason. When I spoke to their supervisor, she explained that she noticed Natalie crying at her station. She didn't want her to think she had to stay at work if she was going through a difficult time, so she offered to let Natalie go home for the day to be supportive.

As I pieced the story together, several different truths became clear. To Natalie, it was true that she was being singled out by her coworker and felt unwelcome. To her coworker, it was true that she didn't know Natalie and had not asked the supervisor to send her home. To her supervisor, it was true that she was just trying to be kind to her employee. Each person experienced a different truth, and each of their truths were very real to them. *The* truth wasn't any particular person's recollection of the events, but pieces and parts from each.

SATYA | TRUTH

I have come to learn that we can't really tell *the* truth; we can only tell *our* truth. Sometimes *the* truth and *our* truth are the same, and sometimes they aren't. Instead of feeling hurt when something seems personal, accepting that *your* truth might not be *the* truth can bring peace. It gives you the space to slow down and consider other possibilities. That was definitely the case for Natalie. Once I explained the others' truths to her, she was able to see the sequence of events more clearly and understand how she had reached the wrong conclusion.

It's easy to assume you've jumped to the right conclusion if you've been right before, but it's important to treat each situation as unique. It comes back to assuming positive intent. You might not understand every detail of a situation, especially if stress is keeping you from considering others' perspectives. Leaving space for possibilities you haven't considered helps tempers un-flare. Assuming positive intent helps you fill in the gaps with healthier possibilities that feel less personal. If you look hard enough, you can even find positive intent behind intentional lies.

When I was maybe five or six, I came home from school one day and told my mom that I needed glasses. I didn't have any trouble seeing things at home, so she was genuinely confused. Being a good mom, she took me to the eye doctor. I failed my exam, got my prescription, and picked out my glasses. I chose a pair that looked just like my grandma's, even though they were wildly out of style. I remember being so excited to show them off at school the next day. It's actually one of my earliest memories. I also remember coming home with a terrible headache. The doctor said it might take my eyes a few days to adjust, but after two weeks my mom realized the real problem: I didn't need glasses at all. In fact, I had 20/20 vision. I just wanted them so badly that I lied to her and the doctor in order to get a pair.

I truly believe that there is a well-intended reason behind every lie, and that reason is usually need- or fear-based. What made getting a pair of glasses so important that I lied several times to multiple people in order to make it happen? It took me almost thirty years to find the answer. Those glasses helped me connect to a family that I didn't feel part of. I grew up in a small house in Austintown, Ohio, with my grandparents, my mom, my aunt, and my cousin. My mom had always been the black sheep of the family, and I extended that title to myself by default. All I wanted was to belong. My grandma and my aunt both had glasses, so childish logic told me that would be a really easy way to fit in. My lie had been need-based. I needed to feel a sense of belonging, so I lied in an effort to create that feeling. While it was self-serving, it was also well-intended.

Fear can drive our lies just as forcefully as needs can. We can lie because we're afraid to admit we've done something wrong and don't want to accept the consequences of our actions. Maybe we lie because we don't want to face an uncomfortable conversation that we know will hurt someone we love. In either instance we are trying to avoid causing harm. While both instances are well-intended, they end up causing harm anyway.

How so? Lying requires more effort than honesty, and that effort becomes a weight for us to bear. The weight of a big lie is obviously much heavier than, say, the weight of telling your kids that Santa Claus exists. With Santa, the joy the lie brings can outweigh the burden of the lie itself. Of course, there's still some harm caused throughout the ruse and once the lie surfaces. While each Christmas is filled with the magic of watching your children's excitement, it's also filled with little bits of guilt to carry from each lie told. And while you don't find many adults that still believe in Santa, there are plenty of us who had to face the disappointment of learning that the people we trust had lied to us.

When a lie comes to light, it breaks trust that may never be repaired. That broken trust can ripple, projecting itself onto other relationships and also impacting them. We might be free from the weight of the lie, but it just gets replaced with the weight of the harm we've caused. Even when we "get away" with a lie, we still carry its weight, thus causing harm to self. Each lie has an Ahimsa cost, and so do some truths. Satya asks us to consider the impact of both our truths and our lies before we act. With the Santa example, every parent has to ask themselves whether the joy of the lie is worth the eventual harm. There is no right answer, and each person's choice looks different based on their values and life experiences.

If you were hoping for some clear guidance in this work, I'm sorry. It's more complex than simple dos and don'ts, and its complexity only increases as we learn more about ourselves. Learning is how we discover our deepest truths, the ones we sometimes lie about to ourselves at first. It requires radical self-honesty, but how do you get honest with yourself? Satya is the essence of intuition, and intuition shows us those deep truths. If you're looking to tap in, go find a coin. Ask a question, flip the coin, and notice your visceral reaction before any thinking happens. You will either be excited that you got what you wanted, or disappointed because you didn't.

The coin flip points you to your want, and your intuition is the feeling of accepting that truth. Let's say I don't know if I want pizza or tacos for dinner (not such a deep truth, but a common conundrum nonetheless). Heads are pizza; tails are tacos. I flip, get heads, and am immediately disappointed. That disappointment leads to a physical reaction. My body slouches forward and I sigh out a short huff of air. That's when I realize that I really want tacos. When I accept that I wanted tacos all along, it feels *right*. That feeling of *right* is intuition, and it also has a physical reaction. My body softens, my shoulders relax, and my brain experiences a sort of *aha* sensation.

If I give myself too much time, I can start talking myself out of the intuition for any number of reasons. If I get pizza, then I have leftovers for lunch the next day, so that's a more efficient option. Maybe I just had tacos yesterday and feel like I should want something different, even though I don't. Intuition is what you feel in that fraction of a second before your brain gets in the way.

If you're anything like me, your brain gets in the way a lot. My brain starts to pull me away from those deeper truths. When I'm veering away from my intuition, I get a "square peg in a round hole" feeling. Something in my life doesn't fit anymore, but I'm trying to force it anyhow. Everything feels like a goddamn struggle! Deep down I know exactly what's wrong, but I'm not ready to listen to my intuition. Maybe what I discovered is difficult or hurtful, or maybe some self-doubt is trickling in. That's when I start lying to myself. For many people, this looks like classic denial: a simple "Oh, that's not true" before ignoring the intuition all together. My brain likes drama, and the lies I tell myself often come dressed as exciting adventures. For example:

My intuition: "You've outgrown your marriage."

My brain, moments later: "No, no, no, that's silly. You have no reason to be unhappy in your marriage. But you know what? It is your heart's deepest desire to get your master's degree overseas. Make it happen."

It might not be classic denial, but it's my brain's way of rejecting my intuition. A friend of mine experiences something similar. She likes to conceptualize large-scale yoga retreat centers or running off to live vanlife when she's avoiding a difficult intuition. My point is, avoiding intuition is not one-size-fits-all denial. These side quests can be super fun to dive into, but if you're entertaining one and life still feels off, you might be ignoring a bigger intuition. The good news is you can still get back to it.

Our deep truths don't disappear, but they do hide. To find them, we have to bring out our inner four-year-old and ask why until we feel satisfied with our answer—until we feel that *right* feeling again. It's important to be honest with yourself during this process, or you'll never reach your truth. There will be moments when you lie to yourself, and that is perfectly normal! I do it constantly. You won't reach that feeling of *right* until you're actually being honest, which just means that you know when you need to keep asking why. Try and be patient with the process, and forgive yourself when you're less than patient. There are important things to learn each time you're wrong along the path to your *right*.

Discovering and living in *your* truth isn't always easy and it isn't always clear, but it does always feel *right*. Practicing Satya can bring deep internal alignment and peace. Sometimes it comes with a cost of temporary hurt or chaos. Deciding whether that cost is worth it is each person's individual truth. All we can do is determine our own truth and respect the truth of others. When you get to know your intuition intimately, it pulls you toward your truths almost effortlessly. Being human becomes less of a struggle and life starts to feel *right*. Truth in all of its complexity leads to harmony.

The Work

Before we dive in, let's start with our temperature check.

How does life feel right now?

1. I feel overwhelmed. Life is coming at me hard and I feel like I can barely keep it together.
2. I feel okay. I have some things I'm working through, and my to-do list is longer than I like it to be. But overall I'm doing fine.
3. I feel great! My heart and mind are wide open, and my stress level is manageable.

Next, find your work:

THE WORK AT OVERWHELMED

Be honest with yourself about how you're feeling. Name the emotions that are coming up.

Let this be enough work for now.

THE WORK AT OKAY

Reflect on a lie you've told, big or small. Was it driven by need, fear, or something else entirely?

Consider the Ahimsa cost (immediate and eventual) of a recent lie you've told.

THE WORK AT GREAT

Practice the coin flip trick to tap into your intuition. Do this as many times as you need to let that feeling of *right* really resonate in your body. Then, pay attention to the times when it happens organically in your life.

Reflect on a time when you jumped to the wrong conclusion. Consider the various facets of truth that were involved, both from your perspective and from others'. How many truths (*yours, theirs,* and *the*) can you identify?

YOUR WORK

Explore Satya on your own. Notice what resonates. Notice the points of resistance. Notice your body's physical reaction as you explore. Let yourself get curious about what comes up.

Asteya - अस्तेय
uh·stay·uh
Non-Stealing

WHEN I WAS FIFTEEN, I GOT MY FIRST JOB AT A roller-skating rink near Youngstown, Ohio. I worked at the snack bar, hosted birthday parties on the weekends, and did mascot work as a roller-skating kangaroo. I've never been one to take myself too seriously, so that gig was right up my alley. One Saturday, there were nine birthday parties to host. One of my coworkers drove us to the grocery store to pick up the cakes, which we always personalized for each child. We carefully piled the cart high and checked out. She pulled her car up front so we could load everything more easily. We did a final cake count and noticed that there were only eight cakes in the car instead of the nine we bought. I looked around to see if we had set one down somewhere while trying to get the others loaded, but there was nothing in sight.

Right then, I noticed a woman walking a little too fast to her car, shifting her gaze from side to side, and piling bags into the front of her cart to cover what was clearly a cake box. It was pretty obvious what had happened. I still can't believe we didn't notice her snatching that cake! I told my coworker what I saw, and in a frustrated huff she slammed the door to her running car, which had all of the other cakes now locked inside. This was not our day. Eventually, the police came to unlock her car, and we drove back to the skating rink and told our boss what happened. I was so nervous and felt certain that we would both be in trouble. Luckily our story just gave everyone a good laugh, which definitely helped lighten the mood. While it didn't turn out to be a big deal, I still remember feeling stressed and angry the rest of that shift.

Stealing doesn't feel good for anyone involved. It hurts the victim because it causes loss, which is always accompanied by a period of grief. Yep, even a stolen cake caused me to experience denial, anger, bargaining, and depression before I reached acceptance. It also disrupts the victim's sense of safety and can create a cycle of self-blame, as was the case for me. Why didn't I notice her taking that cake? In my mind, everything was *my* fault because I hadn't prevented *her* crime. To this day I still get anxious stepping away from my grocery cart.

ASTEYA | NON-STEALING

Stealing doesn't just hurt the victim though. It also hurts the perpetrator via guilt and shaken pride. Guilt after stealing is an expected emotion for most people. Shaken pride, however, is an unintended consequence. It feels better to earn the things we get in life. At first it might be exciting to acquire things we haven't earned, but the satisfaction of *having* is fleeting. We end up with what we wanted, but we aren't proud of how we got it. Asteya asks us to put in the work—to only obtain the things we truly earn.

Most of the time the things we steal aren't actually *things*. How many times have you been at dinner where everyone is glued to their phone, yourself included? Or what about those times when a friend is pouring their heart out, and you're half-listening or just waiting to tell them how they can quickly fix their problem. While it's less apparent than "forgetting" to return your friend's hoodie, a lack of presence is still stealing. It's stealing time from those you love. Our world today has conditioned us to fill every available moment with stimulus, so we usually have a few varieties at the ready when we feel boredom creeping up. Most of the time, having your brain stretched between several different things is fine. I love hanging out with my best friend, scrolling through social media, half-watching some show, talking a bit, and throwing gross old toys for her dogs to fetch. I also know that my recollection during times like that is almost zero. It might not matter if I remember how many computers she has to set up that week, but when the conversation shifts to something deeper, my attention needs to shift with it.

Knowing when and how to become more present is the trick. If you are sensitive to energy, you can usually feel it shift. If you are more analytical, noticing context clues in language and nonverbal behavior can tip you off. However you notice the tone of a conversation change, it is your cue to listen more intentionally. Your thoughts and phone might be fighting for your attention, but if you physically arrange your body toward that person and root your feet to the ground, you immediately become more present. It doesn't mean that your mind won't wander, but those physical actions set you up to really listen. Hundreds of different things fight for our attention all day, so giving someone your focused attention means more now than it ever has before.

Being present during our interactions with others is important in this practice and so is creating a welcoming space for those interactions to authentically exist. In 2019, my friend and I went to a yoga festival. I normally practice vinyasa-style yoga, but when I go to festivals I like to experience things outside of my comfort zone. I'll sign up for chanting classes, forest bathing, ecstatic dance, and basically anything that sounds uncomfortable or unfamiliar. Most of my personal growth has come from discomfort, so I force myself to lean

ASTEYA | NON-STEALING

into it from time to time. At this particular festival, one of the lectures I attended was about spiritual bypassing. Being unfamiliar with the term, I had no idea what to expect, but I was ready for the experience. Well, I thought I was ready.

When I arrived at the class, I noticed the room was filled with mostly black women. Immediately, I thought that I didn't belong. This probably wasn't subject matter that was intended for me, a white woman. I almost left, but then I remembered the importance of discomfort. I also realized that most people of color probably felt the exact same way I did when they walked into a mostly white yoga studio. So I stayed and let myself have the experience. The discussion was uncomfortable for me the whole time, mostly because it challenged my deep-rooted programming to always be uplifting (i.e., "toxic positivity"). There's one moment I'll never forget. A woman near me shared her recent experience at the studio where she practiced. She had been going through one of the most difficult times in her life and desperately needed some time on her mat. Her class ended with a very common closing, "the light and love in me sees and honors the light and love in you." After class, she said she approached the instructor and simply asked if her darkness was welcome there, too.

I'm not sure I heard much else after she spoke. Her words were all I could think about, and their weight was heavy. A piece of her felt excluded when she most needed her whole self to be recognized and accepted. Until that moment,

I always thought that lifting people up when they were down was the most helpful thing you could do. In that room, I realized that true Asteya is holding space for people as they are, not as I want them to be. It is support instead of solutions. It is not stealing from someone's truth by rejecting a part of their experience you'd like to fix. And it is being mindful of the impact of your words and actions.

The same way your words and actions impact others, their words and actions impact you. Enforcing boundaries and fostering a healthy balance in our relationships is how we practice Asteya toward ourselves. Our loved ones need us, and sometimes they need a lot more from us than other times. Our world gets smaller when we're "going through it" (i.e., shit is hitting the fan), and it becomes difficult to focus on anything other than the problems we are facing. At times like this, our loved ones might not realize when they are taking more than we have to give. When that happens, we can choose to kindly set a boundary or give more than we have to offer.

It's easy to give beyond our means. We want to support our loved ones and will often make sacrifices to do so. Of course it's important to give in our relationships, but to give fully we need to respect our individual limits so we aren't pouring from an empty cup. You must allow yourself to replenish so you can stay full. When we keep ourselves full we have the space to experience all that life is offering.

ASTEYA | NON-STEALING

The more fully we can experience life, the more we begin to see our connection to a world larger than our own. When we volunteer our time or upcycle something that was destined for a landfill, we altruistically practice Asteya. The very act of giving back, or not taking beyond our need, is a gesture of service to our world. It is not only non-stealing; it is anti-stealing. Everything we have or do has an external cost. When we work to balance our individual impact, we connect to our greater world and replenish more holistically.

As with all of this work, sometimes you'll give or take too much. Sometimes you won't be as present as you wish you could be, and you might feel like you're getting it wrong. The Yamas don't ask for perfection; they simply ask for awareness. Notice what you are doing versus what you'd like to be doing. Bridge the gaps when you have the capacity, and forgive yourself when you don't. Asteya asks much more of us than to simply not steal tangible things, but its practice offers the richest experience of life in return. When we earn, we are rewarded with pride. When we hold space for others, we connect more authentically. When we set healthy boundaries, we have space to live our fullest lives. And when we replenish our world, we impact others in immeasurable ways. By not stealing, we gain so much more.

The Work

How does life feel right now?

1. I feel overwhelmed. Life is coming at me hard and I feel like I can barely keep it together.
2. I feel okay. I have some things I'm working through, and my to-do list is longer than I like it to be. But overall I'm doing fine.
3. I feel great! My heart and mind are wide open, and my stress level is manageable.

Next, find your work:

THE WORK AT OVERWHELMED

Kindly set a boundary in an area of your life where you don't currently have the capacity to give.

Let this be enough work for now.

THE WORK AT OKAY

Think about something you want and then make a plan to earn it. Once you've earned it, reflect on how you feel.

Reflect on a time when you gave beyond your limit. What feelings did you experience leading up to your limit? After?

THE WORK AT GREAT

Consider ways you can practice anti-stealing. What is the impact of something you have or do, and what actions can you take to help balance that cost? Can you upcycle/repurpose something you'd normally throw away instead of buying new? Maybe you're able to donate to or volunteer at a nonprofit whose mission you're passionate about. What about reducing your food waste or regrowing your veggies? (There are some awesome video tutorials on this!)

When a conversation calls for it, let yourself be fully present and intentionally listen to the other person. Turn your body toward them, root your feet to the ground, and be there. As you become more present during your conversations with others, notice times where you might be stealing from an experience they are sharing with you. Do you interrupt with solutions? Do you gaslight their feelings? Do you one-up their story? Notice your reactions before acting on them. Practice pausing to listen instead of stealing from their experience.

YOUR WORK

Explore Asteya on your own. Notice what resonates. Notice the points of resistance. Notice your body's physical reaction as you explore. Let yourself get curious about what comes up.

Brahmacharya - ब्रह्मचर्य
bra·ma·char·ey·uh
~~Non-excess~~
Enough

REMEMBER THAT BEANIE BABY COLLECTION I mentioned early on? Well, it was more of a problem than a collection. I don't remember exactly how many I had, but it was two large trunks full. One trunk was purple and one was teal. Funny, those are still my two favorite colors. Anyhow, my aunt and cousin (the ones I grew up with) were getting ready for a trip to Hawaii back in the '90s. I was super jealous! We grew up on the lower end of lower-middle-class, so "vacation" wasn't really in our vocabulary. My aunt had worked hard to save up though, and she must have been so proud to be able to make that trip happen.

After they got back, they took their pictures to get developed so we could live vicariously through their adventures (*developing* pictures is what you did back in the day before smartphones, and it was a four-mile walk uphill both ways to the local Walgreens). As we flipped through, I noticed some unexpected yet familiar faces. Two of my Beanie Babies were in most of their pictures! I saw them buried in the sand, wearing goggles by the ocean, and posing with my cousin for a photo shoot. My jaw dropped once I realized she had kidnapped them!

When comprehension crept across my face all she could do was laugh and laugh. "We've had them for MONTHS! You have so many goddamn Beanie Babies you didn't even notice!" she cackled. A different roll of film showed pictures of them at a local Olive Garden and out on a hike. I was pissed! I couldn't believe she had the nerve to steal them and then tell me that I hadn't noticed! Of course, she was right. There was no way I could tell you the specific number of Beanie Babies I had, nor did I even look at or play with any of them. I just had them because everyone else did.

I definitely didn't take her point at my young age, but I was clearly living in a Beanie Baby surplus. It wasn't until I started working with Brahmacharya in teacher training that I started to understand the true impact of excess. The things we own can start to own us, thus perpetuating a dangerous cycle of greed and desire. We don't actually need all that much to get through life, but we do need more than ever before to experience it fully. If you want to get technical, we don't *need* anything other than food, water, clothing, shelter, and safety to *exist*. But to really *live*, we have to add a few things to the list. Probably not one hundred-plus Beanie Babies though. For me, this work has been more about finding the balance of *enough* rather than eliminating all excess.

Most of what we're told we need we really don't. I definitely don't need a phone, a tablet, *and* a laptop. I *do* need a phone and either a tablet or a laptop, but I *don't* need to upgrade them every single year. How can you tell what is an actual need when there are a million wants within those needs waiting to tempt us? At times like this, I like to do a little yogi math when I'm not being impulsive. How much Ahimsa does this want cost? I consider it financially and spatially. Will this hurt my budget or stress me out by cluttering my space? If so, I pass on the purchase. Next, I consider the planet. Do I need this so much that its environmental impact is worth it? Am I replacing something that's actually damaged, or do I just want something shiny and new for no real reason? Those answers always help, and I feel good about my choices after considering them. Do I still have way too many pairs of leggings? Absolutely. But I definitely have less than I would without this work.

Our society ties personal value to how much we have, so of course we're going to want more than we actually need.

Society also ties personal value to how much we do. We're told that the more we have and the more we accomplish, the more worthy we are as a person. Of course, all of that is total bullshit. Here's the thing: People have inherent value regardless of what they have or accomplish. You have inherent value regardless of what you have or accomplish. I have inherent value regardless of what I have or accomplish. I don't feel great when I'm running myself ragged, but I feel like I'm *supposed* to, so I do it all the time. My therapist calls this over-functioning. Whether it's too much work, exercise, introspection, or socializing, living in excess is exhausting. When I'm over-functioning my brain is foggy, I'm tired, and my fuse is really fucking short. I hate feeling that way, and I bet the people I interact with don't love it either.

Excess isn't always doing too much though. Sometimes it's doing too little. In a world that pushes us to always do more, sometimes you will charge forward and burn out. Other times you might shut down entirely rather than fall short of an unachievable expectation. This is still excess, just in the opposite direction. By practicing Brahmacharya, we learn to find our individual quantity of *enough*. Moderation is very personal and nuanced. What is enough for me might be too much for you or vice versa. It all comes down to exploring how you feel compared to how you want to feel in any given moment and taking steps to balance whatever feels off.

I never feel my best on either end of an extreme. I might want to eat an entire pizza, but I know that I will feel sick afterwards if I do. Maybe I want to skip yoga all week when work gets busy, but I know I won't feel mentally or physically great if I don't get to class. It's easy to assume moderation means *less* in a world that is always asking for *more*, but that's not always the case. Moderation means finding that perfect balance of enough, that blissful mix of indulgence and restraint where we feed both our bodies and our souls. I don't just mean *feed* in the dietary sense, but *feed* as it relates to everything we fill ourselves up with. How much work, rest, food, sex, socializing, entertainment, play, spending, saving, inebriation, introspection, and exercise we need is individual. That amount also changes, sometimes as often as day to day. If you keep an open dialogue with yourself, you will start to notice your individual *enough*, and it usually won't be found in the extremes.

Extremes show up everywhere, even in this work. It's common to see most Yamas prefixed with a *non*, meaning *don't*. My ex used to say, "Words have meaning." He usually said it to poke fun at me when I was struggling to articulate something, which happened daily. But he was right, and it's why I chose softer language for most of this work. The thing is, humans won't *always* or *never* behave any certain way, even when we're told we should. We are creatures of habit, and we're also pretty inconsistent. Absolutism doesn't leave a lot of space for being human. When I give myself permission to be inconsistent, I don't struggle against it. I don't beat myself up for not being or doing *enough*, because I know it's not true. This is the very essence of what moderation means to me. I stray, accept it, and gravitate back toward the things that make me feel my best.

When I find balance on my terms, I also find contentment. I know when I have *enough* because I created the definition. Anyone else's definition won't be true for me, and I won't find any contentment there because of that. My definition of *enough* grows as I grow and shows me my new needs when I listen closely. *Enough* feels full but not stuffed. It feels satisfied but not burdened. It feels stimulated but not exhausted. What I need to feel that way is up to me, and what you need to feel that way is up to you.

The Work

How does life feel right now?

1. I feel overwhelmed. Life is coming at me hard and I feel like I can barely keep it together.
2. I feel okay. I have some things I'm working through, and my to-do list is longer than I like it to be. But overall I'm doing fine.
3. I feel great! My heart and mind are wide open, and my stress level is manageable.

Next, find your work:

THE WORK AT OVERWHELMED

Notice any areas of your life where you don't seem to have a balance of *enough*, whether that be too much or too little. Try not to judge or blame; simply notice without any pressure to make changes. The awareness alone will set you up to find balance when you're ready.

Let this be enough work for now.

THE WORK AT OKAY

Do the yogi math on an upcoming want. How much Ahimsa does this want cost (consider self, others, and the Earth)? Am I replacing something that's actually damaged, or do I just want something new? Then decide if the want is worth the cost.

Spend some time listening to your body. Find your *enough* with some common things like work, food, or screen time. How does your body tell you when you've reached *enough*?

THE WORK AT GREAT

Reflect on how you feel emotionally when you are living in excess in a certain area of life. Notice the times you feel satisfied versus when you feel in deficit or surplus.

Explore the reasons you push past *enough* into surplus or deficit.

YOUR WORK

Explore Brahmacharya on your own. Notice what resonates. Notice the points of resistance. Notice your body's physical reaction as you explore. Let yourself get curious about what comes up.

Aparigraha - अपरिग्रह
a·par·ey·gra·ha
~~Non-Attachment~~
Softening Attachments

EVERY SO OFTEN I GET A FIRE UNDER MY ASS AND I decide my life needs a change. Most people don't like change when it blindsides them, and I'm no different. But when I get to create change on my own terms I freaking live for it! In late 2017, this self-imposed change came in the form of a move from Akron to Columbus, Ohio. It wasn't a huge move, but it still scratched my itch.

Just a few months after settling in, I started to feel like I had made a huge mistake. Everything I knew and loved was still up north, or at least that's how it felt. All of my friends were still there, and I had left the first house that had ever truly felt like a home to me. I was still married, and I was embarrassed at the thought of asking my husband to move back after he had just agreed to move away. Instead, I asked him to buy another house in Columbus. That seemed...reasonable? A new attachment would force me to release the old ones, right?

Obviously it doesn't work that way, but we went on our next house hunt anyway. One month and two rejected offers later we were no closer to owning our next home. We kept hitting roadblocks, which I took as a sign that we were being guided in a different direction. That direction could have just been pausing our search, but I decided it meant moving back to Akron after all. While I was still embarrassed that I wanted to move again, I talked to my husband and told him how I was feeling. He said he'd be happy to move back and admitted that he was missing Akron a bit, too. I was so relieved and couldn't wait to get back home. I didn't want to be too impulsive, so I started a job search. Once I found something, we could get ourselves back.

After a few months of looking with no offers, I got discouraged. I overcorrected yet again, and we went back out house hunting in Columbus. This time, we found a place. The sale was relatively smooth, which I took to be *another* sign. This time, the universe was telling me that I was where I was supposed to be and I could settle in. Here's the thing. Everything is a sign and nothing is a sign. We find what we're looking for. If we're looking for signs, we find them. What these signs were really pointing to wasn't the "right" place for me to live. They were pointing to an unresolved attachment I was struggling to release. The reason I struggled so hard was because, deep down, I thought that if I let go of Akron I'd never feel that sense of *home* again. I didn't realize that home didn't just exist in Akron; it existed wherever I built it. Of course, there was no way I could see that in the midst of my frantic gripping from one "sign" to the next.

Since I was subconsciously worried that I had lost that sense of home forever, I was trying to control my life to get that feeling back. Funny thing—the moment we think we have control is the moment we have usually lost it. In less than one year I had tried to move *four* times and succeeded twice. Sometimes life happens and we have to move around, but this was all self-imposed. I had clearly lost control, but you couldn't tell me that. I thought I was just rolling with the signs from the universe.

Attachments usually show up when we are trying to control a person or situation. Just because something worked out as planned once or twice doesn't mean we had control over the outcome. When things work out the way we hope, there are usually many other contributing factors at play. For example, you can get to the airport with two hours to spare and catch your flight without issue. That flight wasn't on schedule because you got there early. You could have arrived early just to have your flight cancelled at the last minute. Our preparations don't entitle us to any particular outcome, but that doesn't mean we should throw our hands in the air and stop trying. We can't control life, but it's still reasonable to prepare.

After preparing, it's important to soften our attachments to those desired outcomes. When we attach to an outcome and things aren't going our way, we can grip. Whether we grip ahold of that original desire and try to force it into existence, or onto some new idea we feel is more achievable, we grip. It's difficult to let go of something we desperately want or have worked hard for, but by holding on so tightly we are giving away our freedom. Our attachments control us; we don't control them. If we are laser-focused on our expectations, we can get blinders to other things happening around us and lose presence. We might even lie to maintain our grip or lose ourselves at the expense of our want. Attachments narrow our world by occupying too much space in our minds.

Attachments themselves can take up a lot of headspace and so can the obsessive thoughts that often accompany them. Those thoughts become a different form of attachment all their own. When I wanted to move back to Akron I was so dead set on the idea that it was all I could think about. I'd rehearse the conversation with my husband in my head until it was basically scripted. I had a huge list of houses saved on multiple realty apps and would ruminate for hours on ways to get where I wanted to go. When I shifted my focus to buying a house in Columbus instead, I repeated the pattern. I'd loosen one grip just to tighten another.

It was difficult to see what was happening in the moment because I thought I was just thoroughly considering an important choice. Important choices definitely require careful thought and planning, but they don't require obsession. It can be hard to understand that difference though. I can tell I've shifted from healthy thought to obsession when my thinking becomes repetitive and unproductive. If I'm paying attention, I can watch myself grip tightly to my thoughts as I repeat them over and over.

This gripping often shows up in our relationships, too. Not just romantic relationships, but with friends and family as well. When we love (or even just like) someone, we form an attachment. These attachments can't really be released, nor should they be. Relationships come with connection, and with connection comes attachment. While that is usually normal and healthy, our attachments in relationships can cross the line into unhealthy without us realizing it. Sometimes the dynamic of a relationship changes, so we try to recreate the original status quo instead of allowing it to evolve. Maybe we become so intertwined with another person that we lose our individual self to maintain the unit.

When this happens, we aren't free and neither are they. That's why it's so important to learn how to soften our attachments. Whether you're gripping ahold of a person, outcome, or thought, the work is the same. It starts by accepting that control is a fantasy. We don't really have it, even when we think we do. Holding that truth requires an abundance of trust that we can catch ourselves even when our wants pass us by. When I doubt my ability to overcome a tough situation or to live without someone dear to me, I take time to reflect. I think about the other times in my life where I've gotten through something that seemed insurmountable. When I remember that it is possible, I also remember that how I am feeling is temporary. Of course it is still difficult, but it won't be this difficult forever. The intensity will fade, and sometimes it will even go away. This helps me experience my emotions without attaching to them.

Relaxing into the flow of life is another way to soften our grip. When I think of flowing water I usually think of a calm, clear river. That peaceful imagery caused me to fight against the idea of "flow" for years. How could I flow when life was so chaotic? It sounded like a bunch of bullshit being fed to me by people who had it easy. After reflecting on the idea again, I realized that most water actually flows pretty aggressively. The ocean, rapids, and waterfalls each embody peace and chaos simultaneously. That's what it means to flow with life. To continue forward, no matter how violently you're being pulled. If you grip while you are being pulled, you'll get hurt by the strength of the opposing forces. But if you allow life to carry you forward with less resistance you'll make it through every patch of rapids you face. You might not be unscathed, but you'll definitely be less scathed.

Practicing Aparigraha doesn't mean that everything will always flow effortlessly in and out of your life. What it will do is help you identify your attachments and notice where you need to soften your grip. When you learn to soften, you help yourself and the people you love feel freedom. Holding on holds us back from experiencing life. Let go when you can, and soften when you can't.

The Work

How does life feel right now?

1. I feel overwhelmed. Life is coming at me hard and I feel like I can barely keep it together.
2. I feel okay. I have some things I'm working through, and my to-do list is longer than I like it to be. But overall I'm doing fine.
3. I feel great! My heart and mind are wide open, and my stress level is manageable.

Next, find your work:

THE WORK AT OVERWHELMED

Identify a thought that you are currently attaching to (something you are overthinking or ruminating on). Take a moment to pause and accept that this is happening without trying to stop the cycle. That's all, just pause and accept it.

Let this be enough work for now.

APARIGRAHA | SOFTENING ATTACHMENTS

THE WORK AT OKAY

Think about a situation you thought you had control over that went as planned. Consider the outside influences that contributed to the outcome.

Reflect on an ending where you gripped more tightly as it was approaching. What was your experience? What about one where you were in flow?

THE WORK AT GREAT

What things, situations, thoughts, or people do you find yourself attaching to in an unhealthy way? What can you do to soften your grip and create more freedom?

Consider an upcoming event that you have to prepare for. Work on preparing without attaching to your desired outcome. Allow the outcome to be whatever it is.

YOUR WORK

Explore Aparigraha on your own. Notice what resonates. Notice the points of resistance. Notice your body's physical reaction as you explore. Let yourself get curious about what comes up.

The Niyamas
nee·yah·muhs

"This is my simple religion. There is no need for temples; no need for complicated philosophy. Our own brain, our own heart is our temple; the philosophy is kindness."
—Dalai Lama

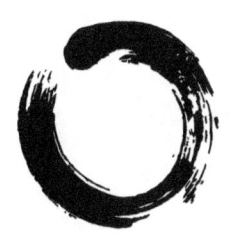

Saucha - शौच
sow·chuh
Purification

OUR INNER WORK STARTS WITH A CLEANSE. No, not a juice cleanse. For the love of God, no more juice cleanses. Saucha is more of a life cleanse.

I've always been a purger. Long before Marie Kondo took the world by storm, I was going through my things once a year and donating anything I hadn't seen or used in that time. Getting rid of shit feels great! What takes up space physically also takes up space mentally, so the things we own can start to own us.

I saw that from a young age by watching my mom. She was always buying *stuff*. Lots and lots of stuff. She wasn't able to work for most of my childhood due to illness. Once she was healthy and able to find a job, any money she earned quickly burned a hole in her pocket. She would buy random things throughout the year and hold onto them as Christmas presents for coworkers she didn't even like. She'd buy clothes that didn't fit her yet as inspiration to eventually shrink into them. This is also definitely how I ended up with all of those damn Beanie Babies!

I have noticed that my childhood shows up in my adult life in two different ways. I've either adopted the habits I learned from the people around me, or I rejected them completely as a means of rebellion. I'm sure there is some middle ground, but those two patterns really stand out. When it comes to *stuff*, I ran the other way.

My childhood home was a stressful place for me. I think that's why I equate *stuff* to stress. To this day, I'm not very productive in a cluttered environment. I get overwhelmed almost immediately when I see an abundance of anything. Boxes, grocery bags to unpack, emails, knickknacks, papers—all of it. Even if it's neatly organized, it just looks like work and I feel burdened by it. I'm not a minimalist, but I also don't have a ton of shit for no reason. My spaces are all carefully created to include things that make me happy and give me room to breathe.

Having tidy spaces is how I keep my environment pure. Sure, they're clean, too. Not obsessively clean, but not dirty by any means. My point is, tidy isn't the only form of environmental purity. It's also not an option for everyone, especially those with kids. I don't have kids, but if I did I'd probably be annoyed by or envious of this section so far. Just like the Yamas, our Niyamas aren't black and white either. Keeping my environment pure has been really important to my mental health, but it's certainly not the only way you can or should practice Saucha.

Purification helps you feel lighter by cleaning up whatever is weighing you down. It's not just *stuff* that can feel heavy. More often it's the things we consume—food, drink, substances, people, activities. Everything we interact with gets "consumed" and becomes a part of us. Those things can help us feel light, or they can become a burden.

Let's start with the things we put into our bodies physically. Saucha and Bramacharya pair well here. I love french fries and nice beer, especially out on a patio. It's one of my absolute favorite treats! If I consumed nothing but french fries and beer, the satisfaction of that experience would be fleeting. I would enjoy it less and less, and I definitely wouldn't feel my best physically for long. If I enjoy it every so often and spend the majority of my time eating nutritiously, I can have the best of both worlds. I get to have the things I love, I still love them because I haven't devalued them by overindulging, and it doesn't negatively impact me because I'm maintaining balance.

Extremes are my quickest path to feeling like a failure. It took years for me to stop guilting myself for eating or drinking something I "shouldn't." Labeling foods as "good" or "bad" was mentally unhealthy and just caused me to spiral. I'm not here to tell you to eat only the cleanest foods, drink only purified water, and never consume alcohol or get high. Yes, the things we put into our bodies become part of us. And yes, it's okay that sometimes those things aren't super pure. Pair your purification and moderation in a way that feels healthy to you. Learn how light it feels to eat and drink in a clean way, and then find your personal balance of *enough* indulgence from there.

Cleaning up the things you consume outside of your body can help you feel even lighter than cleaning up what you put in it. Saucha isn't just about your physical environment; it's also about your mental environment. We don't have a say in everything we consume. The world shoves messaging into our eyes all day long. Unless you live in the middle of the woods free from the burdens of society, it's going to be hard to avoid consuming the hundreds of ads we encounter each day. We can't tell our brains to stop seeing and reading the things that are put in front of us. You *do* have a say in the things you *choose* to see, read, and hear, though. Like, exclusively. That's 100 percent your choice.

Yes, I'm talking about TV, social media, books, the internet, music, video games, and all the other forms of entertainment in your life. Whether it was TV in the '90s or social media now, I've always been told that it's all bad for me and "rots my brain." I'm sure that can be true in some instances, but I don't actually think entertainment is *all* bad. Sometimes consuming something mindless is a necessary escape from life's heaviness. Also, I can choose to consume things that are good for my mental health. I'm not in a constant state of reevaluating every single thing I read or watch, but I do take notice. Is my social media feed funny and inspiring, or are there some accounts in my timeline that cause unhealthy comparison? Is reading the news keeping me informed or sending me down a rabbit hole of hopelessness? What about other entertainment? If everything I'm watching or playing is negative, I start to notice my attitude shifting in that direction, too.

Even exercise and physical activity sometimes need purifying. It might seem counterintuitive for something healthy to become unhealthy, but it happens all the time. How can you tell when something beneficial turns the corner? When something that once was healthy now hurts your mental health, it might be time to clean it up. Activity and exercise can become an obsession, which can start to weigh on us. A healthy mental environment has space for each of the many different things you care about. Purification is about feeling light, not weighed down. If one thing is consuming most of your headspace, it might be holding you back even if it looks healthy on the surface.

This happens all too often with people as well. Relationships are the most difficult and most important part of your life to purify. It's not as easy as simply cutting people out of your life either. We don't always notice toxic behavior, and when we do, sometimes we aren't ready to accept what we've discovered. Oftentimes love is in the way of clarity, so we don't even see how someone is impacting us. Plus, if you always assume positive intent, it's easy to justify another's behavior because you know they mean well. And here's the thing: They usually do mean well. We're all just doing our best with whatever tools we've collected along our journey so far. It's just that sometimes those tools are pretty fucked up and do more harm than good.

It can be so difficult to be objective about the people in our lives. Checking in with myself has really helped me see my relationships more clearly. If I'm feeling down or stressed and there's not a clear cause, I start to examine what I'm consuming—people included. I start by checking who I am when I'm around someone. I ask myself if I like who I am when I'm with them and if I feel safe being my true self. If either answer is no, I take a closer look.

If I don't like who I am around someone, I ask why. Is it because I'm comparing myself to them? If so, are they encouraging that or am I? Do they bring out a side of me I'm working to grow through? If they promote comparison or hold me back from growth, that person might not be healthy for me anymore.

What about being my true self? Do I feel like I have to act a certain way around this person in order for them to like me? Is that true, or just something I've told myself? If I'm not being my true self, sometimes I'm holding myself back from being vulnerable at no fault of their own. That tells me I have some internal work to do. If I'm not being my true self because I have tried before and it was met with judgement or disinterest, that person might not be healthy for me anymore.

Realizing that someone is no longer healthy for you can be difficult to accept. It takes time, and I usually revisit the same questions before the realization lands. Once I learn *and* accept that someone isn't healthy for me anymore, I start creating a little space. I see and talk to them less often and evaluate how that feels. If I feel better, I give myself even more space. Boundaries are healthy, and so is sharing why you need them. Cutting toxic things from your life with a clean break can feel great. Unfollow that account and never look back! It doesn't usually work that way with people, though. Ghosting is a dick move. It might be easier at first, but sharing why you need space brings everyone closure, frees you from the weight of your unspoken words, and creates the opportunity for growth.

Practicing Saucha brings us clarity and lightness. It also brings difficult choices when we discover we need to eliminate things or people that are weighing us down. Just like practicing each Yama looks different at the various stages of life, so does each Niyama. Life has periods of purification and periods of toxicity. It's important to regularly check in with yourself and make shifts toward feeling your lightest.

The Work

How does life feel right now?

1. I feel overwhelmed. Life is coming at me hard and I feel like I can barely keep it together.
2. I feel okay. I have some things I'm working through, and my to-do list is longer than I like it to be. But overall I'm doing fine.
3. I feel great! My heart and mind are wide open, and my stress level is manageable.

Next, find your work:

THE WORK AT OVERWHELMED

Unfollow an account (or twenty) or take a break from trash TV or any other entertainment that makes you feel bad about yourself.

Let this be enough work for now.

THE WORK AT OKAY

Spend time cleaning up a physical space that you've been meaning to get around to. Throw. Shit. Out!

Focus on consuming clean foods and drinks for a while. Reduce or eliminate intoxicants, and see how you feel. Then, see if you can find your own balance of *enough* between clean and indulgence where you still regularly feel light.

THE WORK AT GREAT

Spend one day (or longer) examining the purity of your thoughts. Get honest with yourself about what's coming up, noticing any patterns that might be surfacing. Have you identified any areas of your life that need purifying?

Examine one (or more) of the relationships in your life. Do you like who you are when you are around this person? Is it safe to be your authentic self with them? Explore your answers to see if there is any internal or external work to do.

YOUR WORK

Explore Saucha on your own. Notice what resonates. Notice the points of resistance. Notice your body's physical reaction as you explore. Let yourself get curious about what comes up.

Santosha - सन्तोष
san·tow·shuh
Contentment

I HAVE SPENT MOST OF MY LIFE UNSATISFIED. At least, that's how it felt to me at the time. Any fulfillment I got from my achievements was fleeting, so I'd quickly find something new to pour myself into. Growing up in a lower-income multigenerational household, all I ever wanted was something conventional. To me, that meant a successful career, a stable partner, and a house filled with nice things. After spending years building just that, I felt proud but not satisfied. But that was a good thing, right? I wasn't letting myself get complacent. I didn't spend long questioning why I wasn't content before finding the next thing I wanted to have or do. After all, according to society, the more we have and do, the more value we have as a person, remember?

(Cue dramatic eye roll.)

Contentment doesn't create complacency, but I spent most of my life worrying they were one and the same. I thought I would become complacent if I let myself slow down and feel content for longer than a moment. If I became complacent, I assumed that I would lose everything I had worked so hard for because I lacked the drive to maintain it. Everything would keep moving forward without me as my stillness became stagnation. But contentment doesn't actually equal complacency. Contentment requires consideration and engagement. To feel content, we have to understand what causes our discontent. Complacency on the other hand, is leaning into life without any consideration or engagement whatsoever. As long as you stay connected to your life, complacency can't even show up.

So why wasn't I content? I had considered what I didn't want and taken steps to achieve what I did. I followed the recipe, but the cake was no good. What gives? Somewhere between cracking the eggs and whipping the frosting, I forgot to ask myself if I still even wanted to bake this kind of cake. I just kept baking because I really, *really* wanted that cake when I started. This is how complacency sneaks in. It doesn't show up via contentment; it shows up via disconnection. When I'm disconnected, I end up eating cake I don't even want just because it's there and I put in the work to bake it. When I stay connected to myself,

I know when to toss out the batter before I even bake the damn thing.

Some cakes take a really long time to come together, and we aren't the same person we were when we first started baking. Sometimes we still really want that specific cake, but other times we don't anymore. In this way, contentment and discontentment both tell us our truth. If we are content with something, it feels *right* once we get it. If we aren't, we feel conflicted instead. I tried for years to strong-arm myself into feeling completely content, but it always felt like bullshit. Because it was. I was satisfied with many parts of my life, but not all of them. Take work for example. I have been mostly content with my professional career since it began, but I was unsatisfied in plenty of other areas. That doesn't make my professional satisfaction any less real, and it didn't mean that I was unhappy overall. It just meant that there were other itches left to scratch. I was content and I wasn't content, all at once.

As someone who frequently thinks in absolutes, holding those opposing truths was a struggle. When I said that I've spent most of my life feeling unsatisfied, what I actually meant was that I had never been 100 percent content with every facet of life, which I now realize is pretty normal. Some people say that being happy is a choice. For me that idea was a prison. Applying that concept, if I wasn't happy I was failing because I couldn't get the "choose to be happy" thing right. In reality, I wasn't completely happy because I just wasn't completely happy. Discontentment is a gift. It shows us the areas of our life that we need to reevaluate. If we adopt the "choose to be happy" principle, we are forcing complacency by gaslighting ourselves. Our wants and needs change as we travel down the path of life, so it is normal to be unsatisfied with one aspect or another. Santosha is about enjoying contentment where it exists and exploring the spaces where it doesn't.

We can find contentment in the midst of discontent, too. There is satisfaction in admitting that you are unsatisfied. That headspace has momentum. By accepting your discontent instead of standing still in your denial, you can feel content knowing you are honoring your truth. Every moment of discontent is an opportunity to take a step forward toward happiness. That step might be as small as saying no to plans when we have stretched ourselves too thin. That step is still a step, and it comes with a feeling of empowerment and self-trust. By creating your own life on your own terms, you realize that you have the power to create contentment again when it slips away. So, no—you don't just "choose to be happy" despite life's circumstances. You define what happiness is for you, and then you *create* it. And you can create it again and again whenever its definition changes.

That sense of pride along the path toward contentment turns into peace when you arrive. In most of this work there is no destination. With Santosha, we have to experience a destination to know if we are content there. When we feel completely satisfied, we stop looking for happiness outside of what we currently have. If we find ourselves looking for ways to fill unidentifiable voids, there might be a deeper discontent we need to explore. But there also might not be. Gratitude is the foundation of contentment. Without it, we might never feel satisfied because we don't properly understand how to.

We spend our lives being told that we don't have *enough* and we won't be happy until we obtain whatever it is someone is selling. It's Marketing 101. Once we have that thing, the cycle starts all over again. This makes it difficult to know whether or not we actually are content. Gratitude helps us find our answer. By identifying and appreciating what we love about ourselves and our lives, we realize how much we truly do have. Gratitude lets us define satisfaction on our terms without considering society's or other people's definitions.

Because it is a deeply personal practice, there is no right or wrong way to practice gratitude. My foundation was built by journaling. Each morning, I spent about ten minutes writing down three things I was grateful for. My lists included things like loved ones, character traits about myself, possessions, accomplishments, pets, experiences, professional success, and health. As time went on, I got more and more detailed, narrowing down the reasons behind the initial gratitude. After about two years of regular practice, I felt my perspective on life shift. I started seeing silver linings in challenging circumstances, and I stopped "needing" to shop when I was stressed. Plenty of other specific shifts were happening, too, but mostly life became peaceful in a way I had never felt before. I was finally experiencing contentment.

As with any practice, the more you express gratitude the more it turns into a habit, eventually becoming the lens you use to view the world. Listing the people, possessions, and privileges I was grateful for gave me perspective. That didn't mean I never had new desires or that I wouldn't get upset when life turned into a shitshow. It meant that I knew when I was content because I worked to understand my personal definition of it. A gratitude practice helps us remember the good while facing the difficult. It helps us appreciate the individual things that bring us satisfaction so we don't get lost in larger things we aren't content with yet.

There is no fast pass to satisfaction. Santosha teaches us that we can be content with life while simultaneously wanting more out of it. Feeling discontent because part of our life is out of alignment is different from feeling discontent because we want beyond our need. Contentment isn't one grandiose destination of never-ending happiness, but rather hundreds of smaller, more fleeting ones. Do you know those moments where something really is as great as you imagined it would be? That's contentment. That person who spent years working for something that never quite came together, but they got to watch their child take his first steps, and suddenly they didn't care anymore? That's contentment. What about the times when you get that "wow, life is great" feeling even though you're just sitting around watching Netflix? Yep, that's it, too.

When we define contentment on our own terms via gratitude, we know once we've found it. And when we've found it, we discover the kind of peace that some people spend their lives searching for. Discontentment is part of life. Through this work, we learn whether our discontent is false or actionable. As we live and grow, our needs change. You'll feel the shift and get curious about what it means. When you're outside of your truth, it's hard to feel satisfied. Embrace it. It's just your cue to start exploring. On the other side, there is a whole new level of Santosha that you haven't even experienced yet.

The Work

How does life feel right now?

1. I feel overwhelmed. Life is coming at me hard and I feel like I can barely keep it together.
2. I feel okay. I have some things I'm working through, and my to-do list is longer than I like it to be. But overall I'm doing fine.
3. I feel great! My heart and mind are wide open, and my stress level is manageable.

Next, find your work:

THE WORK AT OVERWHELMED

Each day or so, list three things that you are grateful for. You can write them down, tell them to a loved one, or simply think about them. How you choose to express your gratitude is completely up to you. If you miss a day, let that be okay, but try to keep this up as long as you can.

Let this be enough work for now.

SANTOSHA | CONTENTMENT

THE WORK AT OKAY

Reflect on a time where you achieved/acquired something that you had been working for but didn't feel satisfied with at the end. Why were you unsatisfied?

Expand your gratitude practice. Make an effort to practice daily, and explore why you are identifying the gratitudes you choose. Let your gratitude help you define your contentment.

THE WORK AT GREAT

Consider a part of your life that you are currently unsatisfied with. Can you find a silver lining in your circumstance? Is there an identifiable good mixed in with the bad that can help you find some contentment through the discontent?

How would you define complete contentment in your life right now? If complete contentment is your current experience of life, allow yourself to enjoy that peace. If there are still steps to take toward a greater contentment, what step can you take right now?

YOUR WORK

Explore Santosha on your own. Notice what resonates. Notice the points of resistance. Notice your body's physical reaction as you explore. Let yourself get curious about what comes up.

Tapas - तपस्
ta·pas
Discipline

I HAVE NEVER BEEN VERY DISCIPLINED, AT LEAST not in the traditional sense. I played tennis and volleyball for a couple of years each in school and wasn't very good at either. During my singles matches, I'd sometimes let the other person win because I could tell they wanted it more than I did. In volleyball, my team's drive to win was enough to keep me engaged during our matches, but not enough to get me to practice and improve. I never even got my overhand serve down! Let's not forget band class, which I only joined for the trips. I was the last chair oboe and didn't really practice at home after the first couple of years. I knew I had to be able to play through the music to stay in class and go on the trips, but I knew I didn't have to do much more than that.

Academically, I was originally in honors classes but stopped applying myself to any subject that wasn't English or literature-focused. I barely graduated high school with a two-point-something GPA when all was said and done. Surprisingly, I still got into college. I started off as a journalism major, but soon made the change to marketing. It seemed easy enough, and I figured a business degree might actually get me a job when I graduated. And it did. I started my career in marketing, and that was going the same way as everything else. It was just another thing I was half good at.

I know this all seems contradictory to my need for perfection that I mentioned early on, and it is! Yes, I thought failure was unacceptable, *and* I didn't apply myself diligently to anything. Our subconscious can be self-fulfilling. I felt like a failure, so I found things to reinforce that belief. I'd tell myself that I had to do well and proceed to take no action in that direction, thus fulfilling my prophecy.

One day, I stumbled backwards into an HR career. An old networking contact reached out and talked me into joining her team. I told her plainly that I had no clue what I was doing. She promised to spend time mentoring me, and we went on to work side-by-side for almost seven years. We laughed and cried and argued, sometimes all in the same day. I knew she genuinely believed in me, and she challenged me often because of it.

It was the first time I was more than half good at something. I had done everything up to that point because I thought I should or as a means to an end—nothing because I wanted to. I think we're all familiar with how draining that feeling is. It doesn't mean we shouldn't try things that are suggested to us. In fact, that's exactly why it's so important to try as many things as possible. Saying yes has opened more interesting doors than saying no ever could. I didn't actually *want* to do HR, but I sure as hell didn't want to stay in marketing. So I tried it, I liked it, and I was good at it!

I wasn't good at every single part of the job, but I liked it enough to work on the parts that didn't come naturally. For the first time, I wanted to try harder instead of drifting off to find something different. That feeling is how you learn where to focus your energy. The most rewarding efforts are the ones that bring us a challenge to overcome. We won't always be good at the things that are right for us, but we will always *want* to be. Here, doubt is bound to creep in, and it can stop you in your place if you let it. To overcome doubt, discipline needs to meet desire. Desire without discipline becomes a stagnant cycle of daydreaming. Discipline without desire is just existing without really *living*. When both are in harmony, doubt is simply a small hurdle along the path toward our passions.

Before my HR career, I always wondered why I didn't put much effort into anything, and it left me feeling misdirected. Recently, I was talking to my therapist. I don't even remember what we were talking about, but she said something like, "Oh, well, that probably just wasn't meaningful to you." It was a passive comment, but until that moment I never considered that the things I half-assed weren't meaningful to me. Instead, I reinforced a sense of failure by assuming I wasn't good at them or that I was too lazy to properly apply myself (to be fair, the latter was definitely true sometimes).

Not only did I regularly feel like I was failing, but I also didn't have much self-trust. Since most of my time was spent on things I didn't really enjoy, I'd move onto something new pretty quickly. I didn't trust myself to meet a goal because I never had before. I saw that as another reinforcement of my failures, but that wasn't the case at all. The things I was applying myself to weren't meaningful to me. Or they had been, but weren't any longer.

It is impossible for everything to be important; sometimes things that were important once fall out of favor. When you find something truly meaningful, it will fill you up. You'll find yourself thinking about this new passion, sharing it with your loved ones, and making the time to explore it. Maybe it's not even the activity itself but how you feel after. Take physical activity for example. Getting to the gym is always the hardest part, right? The discipline is arriving and putting in the work, but the reward is that post-workout satisfaction of knowing you're taking care of yourself. Maybe you hate the gym, but you love getting outside for a nice long bike ride. The reward is the same either way. It's just a matter of finding what's meaningful to you.

When you find something that fills you up, having the discipline to work hard at it is how you build self-trust. I've had plenty of "goal weights" and big ideas that never saw the light of day. Missing those marks might have shaken my self-trust, but none of them were actually meaningful to me. I have also had a regular yoga practice for many years, been diligent about saving up to travel, and spent hours learning how to cook. The discipline applied to each of those passions has strengthened my self-trust more than the misses could shake it.

Have there been entire meals that I've had to throw out and trips that were expensive yet underwhelming? Of course. No matter how disciplined we are, we aren't guaranteed the outcomes we hope for. Attaching to expectations keeps us down in our disappointment when things don't turn out how we want. Softening those attachments has helped me see that an unmet expectation doesn't equate to personal failure. There is still value to our discipline even when things don't go to plan. That value becomes clearer the more we detach from our expectations.

This is true of meaningful and conventional disciplines alike. Conventional disciplines aren't very glamorous, which can make redoing work to achieve an outcome a bit more daunting. I'm talking chores, bills, proper nutrition, meeting deadlines, and anything else that feels like an obligation but still adds value to your life. While those aren't the fun stuff, they allow for the fun stuff. Life still requires us to complete tasks that we don't enjoy, and that involves a high level of discipline. Accomplishing those things gives us time to focus on what fills us up while keeping the boring, yet necessary, aspects of our lives afloat.

Conventional disciplines can take up most of our day. Plenty of people work life-sucking jobs in exchange for a paycheck. Those people aren't selling out or settling—we can't all quit our jobs to hike the Appalachian Trail and soul search. That doesn't mean we give up and throw Tapas out the window either. If a part of your life is draining, you can choose to give it less of your energy. We still need to do things we don't enjoy, but we can choose not to attach to them. Detaching means not allowing things that drain us to continue taking up headspace once we finish doing them. When you make that choice, you become more present for the things that truly fill you up.

Life asks a lot of us. Balancing conventional and meaningful disciplines can be overwhelming when we are only considering them from the perspective of work. Perhaps the most important discipline is rest. I can easily become scatterbrained

TAPAS | DISCIPLINE

and focus on a bunch of things I'm half interested in. That gets exhausting. It's also easy to become obsessive about a singular passion. And that gets exhausting. In a society that puts high value on how much we *do*, taking rest almost feels like an act of rebellion.

Rest is more important than any other discipline because it's not celebrated. No one cheers for you when you take a day to yourself because you're feeling overwhelmed. No one celebrates when you ask to be taken off that project that keeps you two hours after work each day. It feels good when others are proud of us, so we tend to focus on the disciplines that produce that result. But when we let ourselves get depleted, there's not much left to give to what we love.

When I stay disciplined in a way that is authentic to my needs I feel fulfilled and motivated. My personal Tapas practice includes specific care routines for my body, mind, and soul. I take care of my body by feeding it nourishing foods, keeping routine medical check-ups, moving it in ways that make me feel alive, and giving myself permission to rest. I take care of my mind through stimulating conversation, going to therapy, focusing my energy on meaningful work, and giving myself permission to rest. I take care of my soul by indulging in my passions, allowing myself to have new experiences, and giving myself permission to rest.

Each Tapas practice is unique, so only *you* can craft your perfect recipe. Just like any great dish, it can take time to exact. You'll know you've got it right when you are accomplishing all of your conventional disciplines while feeling fully present for your meaningful ones. It comes with a sense of pride mixed with the aliveness you feel from feeding your passions. As you grow, so will your needs in this practice. Allowing that shift is a discipline all its own.

TAPAS | DISCIPLINE

The Work

How does life feel right now?

1. I feel overwhelmed. Life is coming at me hard and I feel like I can barely keep it together.
2. I feel okay. I have some things I'm working through, and my to-do list is longer than I like it to be. But overall I'm doing fine.
3. I feel great! My heart and mind are wide open, and my stress level is manageable.

Next, find your work:

THE WORK AT OVERWHELMED

Tackle one conventional discipline that would create unnecessary future stress. Appreciate yourself for crossing it off the list!

Let this be enough work for now.

THE WORK AT OKAY

Give yourself the gift of intentional rest. Schedule and honor it like any other commitment.

Think about a time when you worked hard for something that you earned or accomplished. Now, consider something you got that didn't require much effort. Reflect on the differences between each experience.

THE WORK AT GREAT

What things in your life are currently meaningful to you? Would you like to make more time for them? If so, how can you make that happen while balancing your other necessary disciplines?

Define your personal Tapas practice, taking time to consider mind, body, and soul.

YOUR WORK

Explore Tapas on your own. Notice what resonates. Notice the points of resistance. Notice your body's physical reaction as you explore. Let yourself get curious about what comes up.

Svadhyaya - स्वाध्याय्
svad·yuh·yuh
Self-Study

WE OFTEN TALK ABOUT HOW PEOPLE CHANGE, but I don't think that's quite right. Maybe our children used to love playing with a certain toy that no longer interests them, and that feels like a big shift. Or we run into an old friend at the grocery store, and we notice all of the differences between the person we once knew and the person standing before us now. What feels like change to us is actually growth to them.

Growth is tricky. It sounds like it's going to be linear, but I don't think that's quite right either. Take plants for example. A seed is planted, and it grows up into whatever it's meant to become. But it doesn't just grow *up*. The roots grow down and out to the sides and can get tangled if they run out of space in their pot. The stem breaks through the soil and grows toward the light. Sometimes the plant will move east to west throughout the day as the sun travels across the sky. It might even find something to attach itself to, growing alongside that thing instead of creating its own path. There's not much *up* about it.

The path of self-study is the same. It's the journey of understanding yourself throughout all of your multidirectional growth. The concept of "finding ourselves" is romanticized in films and on social media so frequently that I used to think I needed some grandiose adventure to make the discovery. The truth is, *I* just showed up one day. And I had every day before that, too. I didn't have to run off to *find* myself because I wasn't lost, and neither are you. Connecting to our sense of self is a lifelong conversation, not a singular destination. The more we focus, the deeper that conversation gets.

That focus looks like introspection, and it's why we practice Svadhyaya. When you get curious about yourself, you start to notice the nuances that make you *you*. What do you find yourself doing and why? What are the connections between your emotions and your actions? Why does one thing trigger you when something similar doesn't? The answers to these questions, along with the many others you'll ask, help you understand yourself.

Sometimes the answers you find will make sense, and sometimes they won't. If you stay curious, you will explore

SVADHYAYA | SELF-STUDY

those mysterious parts and grow to understand them as well. This means asking the right questions at the right time. The right question at the wrong time often produces denial and resistance. Right timing paired with the wrong question can lead to misdirection and that feeling of something being off. Here's the fun part of being human: You don't always get the questions or the timing right. Not only that, but the answers to your questions can and frequently will change. That's why there is no destination, because there is always more to discover.

Your Satya practice is a necessary part of self-study, especially during periods of introspection. If the answers you find aren't grounded in truth, they aren't real answers. Trust me, you'll get some wrong along the way. And you should! Wrong points us toward right. When you find a false truth, you won't feel that sense of peace and alignment that an authentic truth brings. That also means it's time to ask some new questions.

Finding your answers is the first step in self-study, but to really connect to ourselves we also have to act on those answers. Shortly after yoga teacher training, I was absolutely certain that I wanted to make teaching yoga my full-time career. I picked up more classes and felt myself gaining momentum toward my goal. Sadly, it didn't take long for teaching to stop feeling like a passion and start feeling like work. My love for the practice was slipping, so I scaled back to teaching just one class per week. Almost overnight, I felt reenergized in the classroom. I realized I didn't want to make teaching yoga my career, no matter how much I *wanted* to want it. I still wanted to teach, just not full-time. Sure, I was wrong about something that once felt very true to me, but acting on my new truth saved me from running full speed ahead toward a destination I didn't actually want to reach.

Staying connected to myself allowed me to accept that new truth with grace. I knew something had shifted. I had the option to either hold on to my original desire or soften my grip and move forward in a more authentic direction. Once I softened, I found peace. Trust me, there are plenty of times when I've gripped instead. When I am prioritizing Svadhyaya, the gripping doesn't feel as necessary. I trust myself because I understand myself. I know I'll make decisions that are in line with my purpose because I've spent time finding it. I trust me to catch me, and I allow my purpose to shift once something no longer feels meaningful. Self-study is a constant conversation, and it is the most important one to have.

The more we understand and connect with ourselves, the better we can empathize when we fall short of our own expectations. In this work, you'll discover things you love about yourself and things you don't. Celebrate the things you love, and celebrate them often! As for the things you don't, start by asking yourself if this is an opportunity for growth or love. If it is an opportunity for growth, work to understand where the belief, behavior, or habit stems from. Understanding creates awareness, and awareness creates the opportunity to pause and choose differently. Remember to find forgiveness along the way. Each of us has work to do, and as we grow we will take steps forward and steps back. Forward isn't "good," and back isn't "bad." Each step is necessary along the path of growth. We are all human, living our own imperfect lives and trying to do a little bit better when we recognize the opportunity.

When our opportunity is one of love instead of growth, the work looks different. We might not have the capacity to prioritize personal growth, or maybe the part of ourselves we don't love isn't something we *should* change (think of societal standards of beauty). Surprisingly, this inner work starts from the outside in. When I'm working to love a part of myself that I currently don't, I flip the mirror around. We are often our harshest critics, so I ask myself if I would love (or at least accept) this "flaw" in someone else. If so, I work to extend that love to myself. If not, my answer might be pointing back to a growth opportunity to explore the root of my judgments.

Life comes with periods of growth, challenge, and stagnation. My challenge and growth periods tend to go hand in hand, and I usually learn the most about myself once I reflect. That's when fun little pieces make their way into the puzzle of my life, and I can see myself a bit more clearly. Sure, it's a two-million-piece puzzle and the cat keeps swatting pieces off the table, down into the air vents, never to be found again. I know it won't ever be finished, but I've grown to love watching it come together in its incomplete imperfection.

This is what reflection feels like, and it's my favorite part of self-study. Each year (sometimes more often), I set aside intentional time to journal and reflect. Writing my thoughts down has always been therapeutic for me, but there are many other ways to reflect as well. Quiet thought, expressive art, supportive conversation, time in nature, and meditation are other productive ways to turn inward. Sometimes when I reflect, I'll notice a span of time where nothing of note really happened. Periods of stillness are part of life, and can be a great time for self-study. While I don't like feeling bored, I try to take advantage of those times to learn more about myself. Reflection, in whichever form and at whichever time, is one of the greatest tools we have to better understand ourselves.

Understanding ourselves is the highest form of self-care we can practice. Bubble baths and mani-pedis are great, but they just scratch the surface. Things, people, and experiences will come and go. They will hold extremely important places in our hearts, and our lives will be even more full because of them. We may have them for a moment or a lifetime, but the one constant we are guaranteed is ourselves. We are all we really have in this life. When I connect to myself and welcome things into my life from that place, the right things find their way to me. Svadhyaya shows me my *meaningful* and unveils gaps in my contentment. It guides me toward my purposes, and as long as I'm staying connected, I'll know if those purposes feel true when I arrive. I am grateful for every person I've met on my journey so far. I am most grateful that I get to spend my entire journey with me, and that I have prioritized understanding and loving myself, just as I am.

The Work

How does life feel right now?

1. I feel overwhelmed. Life is coming at me hard and I feel like I can barely keep it together.
2. I feel okay. I have some things I'm working through, and my to-do list is longer than I like it to be. But overall I'm doing fine.
3. I feel great! My heart and mind are wide open, and my stress level is manageable.

Next, find your work:

THE WORK AT OVERWHELMED

Celebrate a part of yourself that you love. Maybe write it down, tell a close friend, or speak it to yourself in the mirror. However you do it, keep repeating it until it feels comfortable and true instead of awkward.

Let this be enough work for now.

SVADHYAYA | SELF-STUDY

THE WORK AT OKAY

Focus on introspection. Ask yourself questions to gain a better understanding of *you*. When you make different choices throughout your day, or if a feeling bubbles up out of the blue, get curious about it. Why did you make that choice versus another one? Where did that feeling come from? Why do you feel that way?

As you find answers through your introspection, connect to them. Find ways to honor what you discover about you, even if that means setting a boundary to respect your needs or making one small change in your daily routine. Notice how it feels to take care of yourself in this way.

THE WORK AT GREAT

Spend some time reflecting on a specific period in your life. Was this a significant moment in your life or just a particular period that sticks out to you? Pay attention to what you did, how you felt, and how you spent your time. Do you notice any patterns that are still present in your life?

What is something you don't love about yourself? Is it an opportunity for growth or for love? If it is a growth opportunity, work to understand its origin. From there, create awareness when it comes up—see if you can pause and choose differently. If it is an opportunity for love, do the work from the outside in. Would you love or accept this attribute in someone else? If so, turn that love inward. If not, revisit the opportunity for growth.

YOUR WORK

Explore Svadhyaya on your own. Notice what resonates. Notice the points of resistance. Notice your body's physical reaction as you explore. Let yourself get curious about what comes up.

Isvara Pranidhana - ईश्वरप्रणधिान
ish·var·uh pran·ey·don·uh
~~Surrender~~
Acceptance

THROUGHOUT MY LIFE, I'VE HAD BOTH A GREEN thumb and the touch of death. Any time I got a new plant, I didn't know which was going to show up. When I moved into my apartment, my best friend got me a heart-shaped succulent that we joked represented our friendship. That thing eventually rotted in its pot. Luckily, our friendship didn't meet the same fate. As a child, I remember being able to grow just about anything. It didn't matter if it was flowers or food; if I wanted it to thrive, thrive it did.

When I was maybe ten or eleven, I took an outdoor gardening class at a local park. The class was specifically for children, and we each got a raised bed where we planted different veggies and flowers. Let me tell you, my garden was living its best damn life! Everything was super lush, and my veggies were growing like crazy. I was even more excited because we had the option to enter items to be judged at the city's fair at the end of the summer. That year I planned to enter zucchini, cherry tomatoes, and sunflowers.

The first day of the fair finally came. My mom brought me to my garden bright and early to pick the perfect crops for my entries. When we got there, we noticed that the ground was covered in something red. Upon closer inspection, I could tell that it was tons of little tomatoes. Some local kids must have come to the gardens the night before and had a tomato fight. I ran over to my plot, praying that they didn't touch my cherry tomatoes so I could still enter them in the fair. No luck. Every single red tomato had been plucked from my plants; they were now getting even more smooshed beneath my feet. I fucking lost it. I cried and cried until I could barely breathe. I had worked so hard tending my garden all summer just for some little shits to ruin all of my hard work.

After a nice long meltdown, I pulled myself together and accepted what had happened. After all, there was nothing I could do about it. Plus, I still had my zucchini and sunflowers to enter. As I sulked in front of my tomato plants, examining their many unripe green tomatoes, I got an idea. I asked my mom for the regulation book and pulled up the section on cherry tomatoes. It said the judges were looking for ten tomatoes of consistent size, shape, and color. Maybe I didn't have ten red tomatoes, but I sure as hell had ten green ones. I picked the ten most symmetrical unripe tomatoes I could find and submitted them to the fair. Wouldn't you know it—they won third place!

I could have resisted the new cards I had been dealt and given up on the contest all together. It would have been easy to stay down in the disappointment of it all, gripping tightly to what I wished was happening. Instead, after a few hundred tears I accepted it. That acceptance freed me from the weight of my emotions, and I was able to see an opportunity. As with this story, the practices of Aparigraha and Isvara Pranidhana usually go hand in hand. We aren't accepting something if we are trying to control it. Since we can't actually control much, those efforts end up being in vain. Life is going to happen with or without our permission. We can let ourselves be held down by our false sense of control, or give ourselves the gift of acceptance.

As an agnostic, the "give it to God" idea never landed with me. The concepts of faith and surrender were difficult to wrap my head around, no matter how much I envied the peace they brought to others. Over time I have learned to create acceptance internally. When life doesn't go as planned, I remind myself to slow down and accept it. My emotions like to get ahead of me, so that "slow down" part is a critical first step. Slowing down roots me in the present instead of allowing my emotions to pull me forward past what is actually happening into unfounded worry. Only from the present can I truly work on acceptance.

Acceptance is freeing, but it's not always easy, especially when it comes to our relationships. Family, friends, partners, and colleagues make choices and behave in ways we might not understand. It's great if we can talk about what happened to gain understanding. Explanations are wonderful at easing us into acceptance. The problem is that communication is difficult. And it's scary. We don't want to hurt ourselves or someone we care about, so we can hold back the full truth or even lie. Of course, that usually causes more hurt in the long run. We've all seen that play out a time or twelve. Since we won't always get an explanation, how do we find acceptance without one?

After I moved to Columbus, one of my closest friends started to become distant. We'd still text and talk, but it happened less and less often. I could feel her pulling away, and I didn't understand why. She had other friends and family in Columbus, so we could easily continue to see each other almost as often as we had. I would ask if she was okay or if there was anything we needed to talk about, but I'd never get much of a reply. One day I decided I was done not knowing. I pushed hard for an explanation and got a text with some bullshit half-answer in exchange. I also got my number and all of my social media accounts blocked. Yep, even LinkedIn! I was hurt, especially because I knew she wasn't being honest with me. I was also hurt because people are capable of communicating and I felt entitled to answers. It's difficult to accept a situation we don't fully understand, which is why we often search for closure in the unknown. I was holding on to the hope that she'd reach out and we could talk about what really happened. Boy did I grip tightly.

Don't get me wrong, hope can carry us through some very dark times, but it can also keep us in them. The easiest way to tell if hope is truly serving you is to notice where it's *keeping* you. If it's keeping you in the light when the dark wants to swallow you, that is helpful hope. When it's holding you back from the release of letting go, that is the harmful kind. This hope was just keeping me in the hurt.

So how did I eventually accept it? The answer starts with a fun fact about me: I like to think I've moved beyond the experience of difficult emotions. Clearly, as a formally trained yoga teacher, I'm absolved from experiencing fragility and sadness, right? I'm supposed to easily flow with life and let go with grace. Sure, sure. Since I like to deny that I am still human, my first step was to slow down and allow myself to feel how I was feeling. I had to accept my emotions before I could accept the situation. Acceptance doesn't happen in one big sweeping motion. It happens in stages and with small steps in different directions. Mostly, it's just allowing ourselves to feel and accept our emotions and circumstances so they can move through us instead of getting stuck.

Sometimes, in the middle of processing, we find a bit of potential truth we can make peace with. What others do is rarely about us and usually about them. My holding on had nothing to do with my friend, and her isolating had nothing to do with me. People are often struggling with something they can't quite put into words, so they put it into actions instead. Accepting that everything *feels* personal but rarely *is* was where I found peace.

The idea of seamlessly flowing with life sounds lovely until life happens. Of course I want to give my loved ones the gift of an explanation when I've hurt them to help them move toward acceptance. I also want to easily accept those moments where I know I'll never get my own closure. Sometimes life will be that effortless, and sometimes it won't. When it isn't, I know that I first need to slow down so I have space to eventually accept it, whatever *it* is. And I have to accept the situation just as it is. When I try to force life to fit into a nicely wrapped package of my own creation it's a fucking struggle, and one I always lose. Life exists as it is, not as I want it to be.

Acceptance has brought me my truest experience of peace, and embracing it helped me release the fantasy of control. Once I accepted life, I started to live it. My grip softened and the truth stopped being such a prison. Isvara Pranidhana asks us to accept all that life brings, both internally and externally. Accepting our emotions is just as important as accepting our circumstances. Like the rest of this work, sometimes it's easy and sometimes it takes time. That doesn't mean you're doing it wrong; it means you're human. And that is the most important thing to accept.

The Work

How does life feel right now?

1. I feel overwhelmed. Life is coming at me hard and I feel like I can barely keep it together.
2. I feel okay. I have some things I'm working through, and my to-do list is longer than I like it to be. But overall I'm doing fine.
3. I feel great! My heart and mind are wide open, and my stress level is manageable.

Next, find your work:

THE WORK AT OVERWHELMED

Recognize that life feels like too much right now. Are you adding to life's stress by fixating on something outside of your control? If so, can you soften that grip at all? By pausing your racing mind even once, you lighten your mental burden.

Let this be enough work for now.

ISVARA PRANIDHANA | ACCEPTANCE

THE WORK AT OKAY

Notice when you feel worried, anxious, or angry. Can you trace those emotions back to something you're resisting? What other emotions show up when you're resisting?

The next time you're struggling to accept something, whether it be a situation, emotion, or someone else's actions, practice slowing down and accepting it. Take it one step at a time and allow each step to last as long as it needs to. Slow down, pausing any futuristic thoughts. Notice what you need to accept, both internally and externally. Finally, work to accept it just as it is.

THE WORK AT GREAT

Reflect on a past situation that was difficult to accept. Where did the resistance come from?

Can you identify any patterns in your resistance? Is it more challenging for you to accept yourself, unforeseen or uncontrollable circumstances, difficult emotions, or the choices of others?

YOUR WORK

Explore Isvara Pranidhana on your own. Notice what resonates. Notice the points of resistance. Notice your body's physical reaction as you explore. Let yourself get curious about what comes up.

The Beginning

"We are all wonderful, beautiful wrecks. That's what connects us—that we're all broken, all beautifully imperfect."
—Emilio Estevez

I COULD EASILY DEDICATE AN ENTIRE BOOK TO exploring each Yama or Niyama individually and still not scratch the surface. Their depths are immeasurable. That's why I'm always in this work. I've done it, am doing it, and will always be doing it. I'll get something "wrong" the very moment I get something else "right." The definitions of right and wrong will change, and that will drive me crazy before I remember to slow down and accept it. I'll spend months living in excess, and that time will teach me something about myself I never expected to learn. This work will complement and contradict itself simultaneously, all because life is complicated, beautiful, confusing, and gray.

It's important for you to find your own truths along

your personal journey and to keep finding new truths once the old ones no longer resonate. So much of this work is integrated. Just as the practice integrates, it also shifts with the ebbs and flows of life. Your practice will look different when you face a serious illness, when you're in a healthy relationship, when you lose a loved one, when you retire, and during all of life's other big and small moments. It's never linear, and it's never finished.

After everything that happened in 2020, I felt disconnected from my best self. In fact, I felt exactly like an old version of me that I didn't like very much. I was worried I'd never get back to my best because I was still viewing that as a singular destination. The point of this work isn't to find your best self and live there happily ever after. We don't un-grow, even when we feel like we have. While the foundations you build for yourself might sometimes hide below the weight of life, they won't crumble. This practice will catch you; you just have to let it.

This work is here to help you to accept and experience life as it unfolds, no matter the direction. It's here to help you decide how you want to show up in this world, for others and for yourself. To live in all of your imperfectness. And to discover how to know, love, and accept yourself along this journey of being human.

Gratitude

I AM #BLESSED TO HAVE COME ACROSS SO MANY incredible people throughout my life. This offering wouldn't be complete without expressing my gratitude to each of them.

Karis Benner is my very best friend, and her friendship has reshaped my understanding of love. She has been with me from the very first steps of my journey with the Yamas and Niyamas. From reading them to me in the car during a road trip to supporting me when I chose to share this offering, she has been by my side the entire time. I am forever grateful to have you in my life.

Thank you so much to Jadie Riewoldt and Tara Myers, who took the time to read my work and give me honest feedback. We all need cheerleaders and truth tellers in our lives, and I am so fortunate to have found both in each of you. Your suggestions made this a better offering and your support throughout this journey kept me going.

Deep, deep thanks to Tracy Rhinehart. Your soulful passion for each limb of yoga has inspired me since I first stepped foot in your classroom. I am beyond grateful to have been guided by you throughout my teacher training experience. None of this work is without your influence.

Thank you to Shelly Fink and Beth Paradise. You have both been incredible bosses and even better friends. Shelly, our friendship has shaped so much of who I am, and I certainly wouldn't be here without having known you. And Beth, thank you for all of the grace you have extended me and for making the most difficult time in my life more manageable through your kindness.

Lastly, a thank you to me. No matter how awkward it feels to write this bit of gratitude, I try to practice what I preach. So I'm celebrating my damn self! I wouldn't be here without my people, and I also wouldn't be here without me. I am grateful for my dedication to push through the countless hours of tears and doubt that went into this offering. There are many things in life that don't have an ending, but I also leave a lot undone. This book is one of the few things I have ever wanted to finish, and I am thankful to have given myself that gift.

About the Author

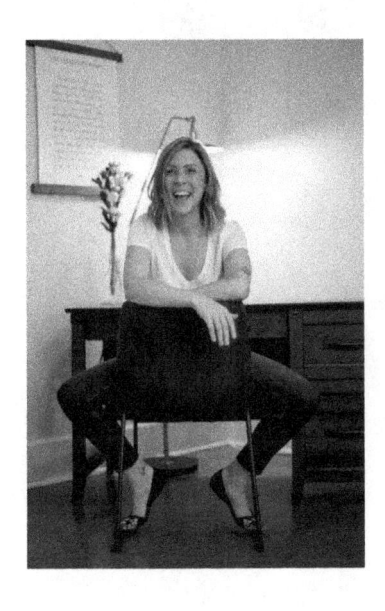

SARA ADAMS enjoys cooking healthy food while simultaneously drinking too much. She doesn't spend excessively, yet opts for lavish nail art when getting manicures. She is an incredible listener who is horribly impatient. She has a least favorite part of her body, even though she'll tell you that you should love every part of yourself. She enjoys new experiences but fears the unknown. She is an imperfect human, just like you.

www.BeingHuman.yoga
www.instagram.com/beinghuman.yoga